ICU Survival Guide

Essential Strategies for Thriving in Critical Care

John T. Dorsett, MD
Critical Care Specialist

Copyright © 2024 by John T. Dorsett, MD. All rights reserved.

No part of this publication may be reproduced, distributed, or transmitted in any form or by any means, including photocopying, recording, or other electronic or mechanical methods, without the prior written permission of the publisher, except in the case of brief quotations embodied in critical reviews and certain other noncommercial uses permitted by copyright law.

Acknowledgements

I would like to extend my sincere gratitude to all those who contributed to the development of this guide. Special thanks to my colleagues, mentors, and the healthcare professionals in critical care who provided their expertise and insights. I am also deeply appreciative of my family for their unwavering support throughout this project. Finally, I would like to acknowledge the editorial and publishing teams for their dedication in bringing this work to fruition.

Preface

The ICU environment is a high-pressure, fast-paced setting that demands precision, prompt decision-making, and multi-disciplinary collaboration. In this ICU Survival Guide: Essential Strategies for Thriving in Critical Care, we aim to provide healthcare professionals, from students to experienced clinicians, with a comprehensive, evidence-based framework to navigate the complexities of critical care. This guide distills essential concepts, protocols, and practices into digestible insights, ensuring healthcare workers are equipped to provide high-quality care under the most challenging circumstances.

Critical care often involves complex, life-altering decisions made under intense pressure, where each action has profound implications. With its in-depth discussion on ICU protocols, critical care management strategies, and common conditions encountered in the unit, this guide serves as a critical resource for both those new to the ICU and seasoned practitioners aiming to refine their skills. By offering a detailed overview of day-to-day operations, from consultations and documentation to advanced sepsis management and mechanical ventilation, this guide empowers healthcare professionals to improve patient outcomes and thrive in this demanding field.

Each chapter in this guide is structured to address pivotal aspects of ICU care. Chapter 1 introduces day and night expectations in the

Medical ICU (MICU), focusing on procedural accuracy, documentation, communication, and interdisciplinary collaboration. These foundational principles ensure that critical care teams operate efficiently and with a clear understanding of responsibilities. Chapter 2 builds on this with a comprehensive exploration of mechanical ventilation, respiratory failure, ARDS management, and more, providing clinicians with the knowledge needed to manage respiratory crises in the ICU. Chapter 3 delves into complex metabolic and acid-base disorders, such as Diabetic Ketoacidosis (DKA) and Hyperosmolar Hyperglycemic State (HHS), along with diagnostic and treatment protocols that are essential for timely and accurate interventions.

The following chapters continue to build expertise, tackling subjects like delirium in the ICU, sedation practices, and the management of ICU drips used for analgesia, sedation, and cardiovascular support. Each section provides actionable insights based on the latest clinical evidence, allowing healthcare professionals to understand both the theoretical underpinnings and practical approaches needed in the ICU setting.

Our approach is rooted in a philosophy of holistic, patient-centered care. Critical care medicine is not solely about managing clinical complications; it also requires emotional intelligence, collaboration, and a commitment to ongoing learning. This guide emphasizes the importance of clear communication with patients' families, interdisciplinary team coordination, and the recognition of subtle but crucial changes in patient status.

In the fast-paced and often overwhelming environment of the ICU, it is easy to become consumed by the urgency of patient care. However, adopting a structured approach, guided by best practices and evidence, ensures that each patient receives the most effective and compassionate care. Through practical protocols, expert insights, and case-based learning, ICU Survival Guide offers an invaluable resource for those seeking to not only survive but excel in critical care.

Whether you are a medical student, a resident, or an experienced intensivist, this guide will serve as a crucial companion on your journey through the complex landscape of ICU medicine. With the right tools, mindset, and strategies, thriving in critical care is not only achievable but inevitable.

John T. Dorsett, MD,
Critical Care Specialist

Acknowledgements

Preface

Table of contents

List of Abbreviations

Table of contents

Chapter 1: Day and Night MICU Expectations

1.1 Consultations

1.2 Patient Readmission

1.3 Documentation

1.4 Transfers

1.5 Summaries and Death Documentation

1.6 Notifications

1.7 Procedures

1.8 Interdisciplinary Conferences

Chapter 2: Comprehensive Overview of Critical Topics in ICU and Pulmonary Medicine

2.1 Mechanical Ventilation

2.2 Respiratory Failure and ARDS Management

2.3 Chronic Obstructive Pulmonary Disease (COPD)

2.4 Asthma Management

2.5 GI Bleeding in the ICU

Chapter 3: Diabetic Ketoacidosis (DKA) and Hyperosmolar Hyperglycemic State (HHS)

3.1 Diagnostic Criteria

3.2 Management of DKA and HHS

3.3 Approach to Acid/Base Disorders

Chapter 4: Sedation in ICU

4.1 Goals of Sedation

4.2 Pharmacological Options

Chapter 5: Delirium in Critical Care

5.1 Definition and Characteristics

5.2 Impact of ICU Delirium

5.3 Risk Factors

5.4 Monitoring Tools

5.5 Management Approaches

List of Abbreviations

ABG - Arterial Blood Gas

APRV - Airway Pressure Release Ventilation

ARDS - Acute Respiratory Distress Syndrome

CAT - COPD Assessment Test

CNS - Central Nervous System

COPD - Chronic Obstructive Pulmonary Disease

CVC - Central Venous Catheter

EDRS - Electronic Death Registration System

EKG - Electrocardiogram

FiO$_2$ - Fraction of Inspired Oxygen

GI - Gastrointestinal

H&P - History and Physical

HHS - Hyperosmolar Hyperglycemic State

ICU - Intensive Care Unit

IBW - Ideal Body Weight

LAMA - Long-Acting Muscarinic Antagonist

LABA - Long-Acting Beta Agonist
MAP - Mean Arterial Pressure
MICU - Medical Intensive Care Unit
NIV - Non-Invasive Ventilation
PAO$_2$ - Partial Pressure of Oxygen in Arterial Blood
PAC - Pressure Assist-Control
PEEP - Positive End-Expiratory Pressure
PSV - Pressure Support Ventilation
SBT - Spontaneous Breathing Trial
SIRS - Systemic Inflammatory Response Syndrome
SOFA - Sepsis-Related Organ Failure Assessment
VSV - Volume Support Ventilation
VTE - Venous Thromboembolism

Chapter 1
Day MICU Expectations

1. Consultations:

Confirm that a consultation order has been placed in the electronic medical records system (e.g., EPIC).

Ensure all consultations are evaluated within 30 minutes.

Present completed consultations to the Fellow or Attending physician.

2. Patient Readmission:

Readmissions to the ICU are considered "bounce backs" if the same Attending or Fellow is on duty.

3. Documentation:

For ICU admissions, a History and Physical (H&P) note is required.

If ICU admission is unnecessary, document findings in a consult note.

4. Transfers:

External transfers should be admitted under the accepting physician's name.

Stable patients transferring to the hospitalist service require coordination with the MAR (Medical Administrative Resident) for team and attending assignment.

The Fellow must directly communicate with the accepting hospitalist.

ICU Residents should provide sign-outs to the receiving team resident.

5. Summaries and Death Documentation:

For patients in the ICU for over 48 hours, prepare a transfer summary.

Document deaths in the system promptly, including an EDRS (Electronic Death Registration System) entry.

6. Notifications:

Notify the Fellow or Attending about critical changes, including new hemodynamic instability, complications from procedures, changes in care goals, or death, followed by a family update.

7. Procedures:

Conduct timeouts before all procedures.

For central venous catheters (CVCs), confirm placement using manometry or transducing before dilation.

Obtain consent for non-emergency procedures and document each procedure.

8. Interdisciplinary Conferences:

Participation in MICU interdisciplinary meetings is mandatory unless patient care requires attention.

Night MICU Expectations

1. Consultations:

Verify that a consultation order has been entered in EPIC.

Residents should present all consultations to the Fellow, regardless of the diagnosis.

2. Notifications:

Inform the Fellow of significant events, including changes in care goals, hemodynamic instability, procedural complications, or death, followed by a family update.

3. Bounce Backs:

Bounce-back guidelines apply at night.

4. Admissions:

The MICU on-call team handles most admissions but may allocate cases to non-call teams to maintain a balanced workload.

5. Ventilator Management:

Changes to ventilator settings must be communicated to the Fellow and Respiratory Therapist (RT).

Do not modify ventilator settings without prior notification to the RT and ICU Fellow.

Sepsis Management

Key Definitions

1. Systemic Inflammatory Response Syndrome (SIRS): Diagnosed with ≥2 of the following:

Abnormal white blood cell count (Leukocytosis >12,000 or <4,000, or Bandemia).

Fever >100.4°F or Hypothermia <96.8°F.

Tachypnea >20 breaths/min.

Tachycardia >90 bpm.

2. Sepsis: SIRS + suspected infection.

3. Severe Sepsis: Sepsis + evidence of organ dysfunction.

4. Septic Shock: Severe sepsis + persistent hypotension despite fluid resuscitation or requiring vasopressors.

SOFA Criteria

Reference: Singer et al., JAMA, 2016.

Treatment Protocols

Fluid Resuscitation:

Administer 30 mL/kg body weight crystalloid fluids promptly.

Place central or arterial lines for hemodynamic instability as needed.

Antibiotics:

Start early with appropriate broad-spectrum coverage (e.g., Vancomycin, Zosyn).

Culture blood, sputum, and urine before initiating therapy.

Vasopressors:

Start norepinephrine if MAP <65 mmHg after fluids.

Consider adding vasopressin or epinephrine for additional support.

Vitamin C, Steroids, and Thiamine:

Emerging data supports adjunctive therapy with these agents to reduce mortality.

Respiratory Failure and ARDS Management

Criteria and Diagnostics:

Hypoxemia (PaO2 <60 mmHg) or Hypercapnia (PaCO2 >45 mmHg).

Confirm with CXR and ABG.

ARDS (Berlin Criteria):

PaO2/FiO2 <300 (mild), <200 (moderate), <100 (severe).

Low tidal volume ventilation (4-6 mL/kg IBW).

Consider prone positioning and ECMO for refractory cases.

References

1. Singer, M., Deutschman, C.S., et al. JAMA, 2016.

2. Marik, P.E., et al. Chest, 2017.

3. Annane, D., et al. NEJM, 2018.

4. Kallet, R.H., et al. Critical Care Medicine, 2005.

Chapter 2
Comprehensive Overview of Critical Topics in ICU and Pulmonary Medicine

Mechanical Ventilation

Mechanical ventilation is a cornerstone of care in the ICU. This guide outlines its critical principles and modes, with evidence-based insights.

Oxygenation Control: Adjusted via Positive End-Expiratory Pressure (PEEP) and Fraction of Inspired Oxygen (FiO2).
Carbon Dioxide (CO2) Control: Managed through Respiratory Rate (RR) and Tidal Volume (TV).

1. Volume Assist-Control (VAC):

Requires pre-setting the respiratory rate and tidal volume.

Patients can initiate additional breaths, with the ventilator delivering the set tidal volume.

Plateau Pressure: Reflects alveolar distension; keep it below 30 cm H_2O for safety.

2. Pressure Assist-Control (PAC):

Sets the respiratory rate and pressure control level.

Inspiratory Time (I-Time): Defines the duration of pressure application during inspiration, influencing the I:E ratio (typically 1:2–1:4).

Ensure the I:E ratio matches the patient's respiratory needs.

3. Pressure Support Ventilation (PSV):

Requires setting pressure support and PEEP.

Facilitates spontaneous breathing, relying on the patient's respiratory drive.

Delivered pressure depends on lung compliance, resulting in variable tidal volumes.

4. Volume Support Ventilation (VSV):

Tidal volume and PEEP are pre-set, and pressure supports auto-adjusts to achieve the desired tidal volume.

Allows for spontaneous breathing.

5. Airway Pressure Release Ventilation (APRV):

Inverse-ratio high-pressure mode enabling spontaneous breathing at elevated lung volumes.

Often used as a "rescue" strategy for refractory cases. Adequate sedation is necessary to prevent patient-ventilator dyssynchrony.

Common Vent Settings:

Tidal Volume (non-ARDS): 6–10 mL/kg Ideal Body Weight (IBW).

PEEP: 5–20 cm H_2O.

Phigh: 20–30 cm H_2O (minor adjustments significantly impact gas exchange).

Thigh: 3–6 seconds (increment by 0.5 seconds as needed).

Tlow: 0.4–0.8 seconds (adjust in 0.1-second increments based on ABG results).

Liberation from Ventilation:

Criteria for weaning include:

Reversal of respiratory failure.

Strong cough reflex.

Clear mentation.

Minimal secretions.

A Spontaneous Breathing Trial (SBT), typically lasting 30–120 minutes on minimal support (e.g., PSV or CPAP), assesses readiness for extubation. Success is indicated by RSBI < 105.

Chronic Obstructive Pulmonary Disease (COPD)

Outpatient Management: Management stratified by exacerbation history and COPD Assessment Test (CAT) score:

Group A: SABA.

Group B: LABA or LAMA.

Group C: LABA + LAMA.

Group D: LABA + LAMA + ICS.

Acute Exacerbations:

Symptoms: Increased sputum, dyspnea, wheezing, tachypnea, and tachycardia.

Labs: CBC, CMP, ABG, CXR, Respiratory Panel.

Treatment includes:

Bronchodilators: Albuterol (2.5 mg q2h) ± Ipratropium.

Steroids: Prednisone 40 mg x 5 days.

Antibiotics: Tailored based on pseudomonas risk and local antibiograms.

Ventilatory Support:

Non-invasive ventilation (NIV): Indicated for hypercapnia and pH > 7.2.

Mechanical Ventilation: Required for refractory acidosis (pH < 7.2).

Asthma Management

Outpatient Therapy:

Stepwise Approach: Escalation from SABA monotherapy to ICS ± LABA, with consideration of biologics (e.g., Omalizumab) in severe cases.

Monitoring: Continuous assessment of oxygenation, RR, and cardiac status.

Acute Exacerbation:

Bronchodilators: Nebulized Albuterol (2.5 mg q2h) ± Ipratropium.

Steroids: Prednisone 40 mg x 5 days.

Intubation/NIV: For severe acidosis (pH < 7.2) or refractory symptoms.

GI Bleeding in the ICU

Differential Diagnoses:

Upper GI Bleeds: Peptic ulcers, varices, Mallory-Weiss tears, malignancy.

Lower GI Bleeds: Diverticulosis, colitis, hemorrhoids, malignancy.

Initial Management:

Resuscitation: Establish IV access with large-bore catheters, initiate fluid and RBC transfusions.

Diagnostics: NG lavage to localize bleeding source.

Pharmacologic Therapy: IV Pantoprazole (80 mg bolus, 8 mg/hour infusion). For variceal bleeds, consider Octreotide.

Consultation: Involve GI, surgery, and interventional radiology as needed.

Transfusion Targets:

Hemoglobin > 7 g/dL for mild bleeds; higher thresholds for active hemorrhage or shock.

References

1. Dodd JW et al., Thorax, 2011.

2. Dodd JW et al., COPD, 2012.

3. ARDS Network, N Engl J Med, 2000.

4. Feinman M, Haut ER, Surg Clin North Am, 2014.

5. Ghassemi KA, Jensen DM, Curr Gastroenterol Rep, 2013.

Chapter 3
Diabetic Ketoacidosis (DKA) and Hyperosmolar Hyperglycemic State (HHS)

Diagnostic Criteria

DKA:

1. Blood glucose > 250 mg/dL (cases of euglycemic DKA have been documented).

2. pH < 7.3 with an elevated anion gap not attributable to other conditions.

3. Serum bicarbonate < 20 mEq/L.

4. Urine ketones, acetone, and beta-hydroxybutyrate (BHB) > 2.

HHS:

1. Blood glucose > 600 mg/dL and serum osmolality > 320 mOsm/L.

2. pH > 7.3.

3. Serum bicarbonate > 20 mEq/L.

Management of DKA and HHS

1. Fluid Resuscitation:

Initiate aggressive fluid replacement immediately, targeting rehydration over 24 hours.

Use isotonic saline initially to expand extracellular volume, then transition to half-normal saline once volume is restored.

Potassium chloride (KCl) supplementation may be required if serum potassium is between 3.3 and 5.0 mEq/L.

If potassium levels fall below 3.3 mEq/L, hold insulin therapy until corrected.

2. Insulin Therapy:

Start insulin drip to halt lipolysis and reduce hepatic keto acid production.

Loading dose: 0.1–0.15 units/kg IV followed by a continuous infusion. Adjust the rate to lower blood glucose by 70–100 mg/dL per hour.

When glucose drops below 200 mg/dL, switch to IV glucose (e.g., D5 ½ NS).

3. Electrolyte Monitoring and Replacement:

Regularly monitor potassium and phosphorus levels (e.g., BMP every 4 hours).

Close the anion gap before transitioning to subcutaneous insulin (e.g., Lantus) with an overlap of two hours with the insulin drip.

Reference:

Gosmanov, A.R., Gosmanova, E.O., & Dillard-Cannon, E. (2014). Management of adult diabetic ketoacidosis. Diabetes, Metabolic Syndrome and Obesity: Targets and Therapy, 7, 255.

Approach to Acid/Base Disorders

1. Step 1: Internal Consistency of ABG:

Analyze pH, $PaCO_2$, and HCO_3 to identify primary disorders (aligned with the pH direction).

2. Step 2: Calculate Anion Gap (AG):

Formula: $Na^+ - (Cl^- + HCO_3^-)$.

Normal AG: ~12.

Primary AG Metabolic Acidosis: AG > 12.

Non-AG Metabolic Acidosis: AG < 12, HCO_3 < 24.

3. Step 3: AG Appropriateness for HCO_3:

> 30: Primary metabolic alkalosis.

24–30: No additional disturbances.

<24: Primary non-AG metabolic acidosis.

4. Step 4: $PaCO_2$ Appropriateness for HCO_3:

Expected $PaCO_2 = 1.5 \times HCO_3 + 8$.

Deviations indicate respiratory compensation or concomitant respiratory acidosis/alkalosis.

Compensatory Equations:

Metabolic Alkalosis: $PaCO_2$ ↑ by 0.7 for each 1 mEq/L increase in HCO_3.

Respiratory Acidosis: Acute: HCO_3 ↑ by 1 per 10 mmHg ↑ in CO_2. Chronic: HCO_3 ↑ by 3.5 per 10 mmHg ↑ in CO_2.

Respiratory Alkalosis: Acute: HCO_3 ↓ by 2 per 10 mmHg ↓ in CO_2. Chronic: HCO_3 ↓ by 5 per 10 mmHg ↓ in CO_2.

Sedation in ICU

Goals:

1. Minimize anxiety and agitation.

2. Optimize patient-ventilator synchrony.

3. Facilitate nursing care and physical therapy.

4. Avoid complications such as prolonged ICU stays, mechanical ventilation, or delirium.

Pharmacological Options

1. Benzodiazepines:

Bind to GABA receptors. Provide sedation, amnesia, anxiolysis, and muscle relaxation.

Common Agents:

Diazepam (Valium): Rapid onset, long half-life. Use in alcohol withdrawal/seizures.

Lorazepam (Ativan): Good for prolonged sedation; risk of oversedation with delayed response.

Midazolam (Versed): Short-term sedation; avoid long infusions due to active metabolite accumulation.

2. Propofol:

Rapid onset with titratable dosing. Suitable for mechanically ventilated patients.

Side effects: Hypotension, bradycardia, triglyceride elevation, rare infusion syndrome.

3. Antipsychotics:

Haloperidol: Controls agitation with minimal respiratory effects. Watch for QT prolongation.

Atypical Antipsychotics (e.g., Quetiapine, Ziprasidone): Fewer side effects, useful for ICU delirium.

4. Dexmedetomidine (Precedex):

Allows interactive sedation with minimal respiratory depression. Risk of bradycardia and hypotension.

5. Ketamine:

Effective for analgesia and sedation, maintaining respiratory drive. Use with caution in renal/hepatic impairment.

6. Adjuncts:

Acetaminophen, NSAIDs, and antiepileptics complement sedation and analgesia regimens.

Chapter 4
Delirium in Critical Care

Definition and Characteristics

Delirium is a neurocognitive disorder marked by:

1. Impaired Attention and Awareness: Reduced ability to concentrate, focus, sustain, or shift attention.

2. Cognitive Changes: Memory deficits, disorientation, language issues, or perceptual disturbances unrelated to preexisting or developing dementia.

3. Rapid Onset and Fluctuation: Symptoms emerge over hours to days and can vary throughout the day.

4. Underlying Causes: Evidence links delirium to medical conditions, substance use, medications, or a combination of these.

5. Critical Illness Association: In ICU patients, delirium may arise from various precipitating or predisposing factors. While reversible, it can lead to long-term cognitive impairments.

Impact of ICU Delirium

Delirium in ICU settings is associated with:

Prolonged mechanical ventilation.

Extended hospital stays.

Increased self-extubation incidents.

Higher mortality rates.

Potential long-term cognitive deficits.

Risk Factors

Medical Conditions: Infections, metabolic disturbances (e.g., renal or liver failure, electrolyte imbalances), hypoxia, CNS pathology, or trauma.

Nutritional Deficiencies: Deficiency of vitamin B12, thiamine, folate, or niacin.

Withdrawal Syndromes: Alcohol or sedative withdrawal.

Endocrine Disorders: Hyper- or hypothyroidism.

Toxins and Heavy Metals: Exposure to environmental or iatrogenic toxins.

Monitoring Tools

1. Richmond Agitation-Sedation Scale (RASS): Used to assess levels of sedation and agitation.

2. Confusion Assessment Method for the ICU (CAM-ICU): A rapid, validated tool with high

sensitivity and specificity for identifying ICU delirium.

Management Approaches

1. Non-Pharmacological Interventions

Orientation and Reorientation: Frequently reorient the patient to time, place, and situation.

Early Mobilization: Encourage physical activity as tolerated.

Sleep-Wake Regulation: Optimize natural cycles using lighting and noise control.

Environment Control: Maintain comfortable temperature, noise, and humidity levels.

Basic Needs: Manage hunger, hydration, bowel, and bladder needs; ensure access to hearing aids and eyeglasses.

Minimize Restraints: Remove catheters or restraints promptly.

Pre-Procedural Explanation: Prepare patients with explanations and proactive pain management.

Stimulation and Engagement: Encourage family visits, provide entertainment, and offer spiritual support.

Cognitive and Relaxation Techniques: Employ behavioral therapy and relaxation practices.

2. Pharmacological Interventions

Pain Control and Correction of Underlying Causes:

Use appropriate analgesics.

Treat infections with antibiotics and address metabolic or micronutrient deficiencies.

Sedation Therapy:

1. Dexmedetomidine: Preferred for sedation with minimal respiratory suppression.

2. Propofol: Effective for short-term sedation in ventilated patients.

3. Avoid Benzodiazepines: Use only for alcohol withdrawal.

Antipsychotics:

Haloperidol: A dopamine (D2) receptor antagonist.

Dose: 2–10 mg IV every 6 hours.

Adverse Effects: Extrapyramidal symptoms (e.g., dystonia, akathisia), QT prolongation, and neuroleptic malignant syndrome.

Atypical Antipsychotics: Alternative agents with fewer extrapyramidal side effects.

Olanzapine:

Dose: Start with 5–10 mg daily; adjust by 5 mg/day as needed, up to 20 mg/day.

Adverse Effects: Orthostatic hypotension, hyperglycemia, QT prolongation, anticholinergic effects.

Quetiapine:

Dose: Start with 50 mg every 12 hours; increase to 400 mg/day as needed.

Note: Dose reduction in hepatic impairment.

References

Zalieckas, J., & Weldon, C. (2015). Sedation and analgesia in the ICU. Seminars in Pediatric Surgery, 24(1), 37-46.

Chapter 5
Common ICU Drips: A Professional Overview

Sedatives, Analgesics, and Paralytics

1. Propofol

Propofol is administered at a standard concentration of 1000 mg/100 mL, with an initial rate of 10 mcg/kg/min, increasing to a maximum of 60 mcg/kg/min. It has a rapid onset and quick recovery profile but may accumulate with prolonged use, leading to extended effects. Propofol Infusion Syndrome, a severe condition with high mortality, can develop within a few days of use.

2. Fentanyl

With a standard concentration of 50 mcg/mL, fentanyl is typically started at 25 mcg/hr and can be titrated up to 300 mcg/hr. It is the preferred analgesic in ICU settings due to its lack of dose adjustments for renal or hepatic dysfunction.

3. Dexmedetomidine

This presynaptic alpha-2 agonist is commonly used for sedation in ICU patients. At a standard concentration of 4 mcg/mL, it starts at 0.2 mcg/kg/hr and can be titrated up to 1.5 mcg/kg/hr. It has a favorable side-effect profile and is suitable for patients not requiring mechanical ventilation.

4. Midazolam

Midazolam, a widely used sedative, is prepared at a concentration of 1 mg/mL and initiated at 1 mg/hr, with a maximum rate of 20 mg/hr. While no specific adjustments are needed for renal or hepatic dysfunction, caution is advised during administration.

5. Cisatracurium

Administered at a concentration of 1 mg/mL, the initial rate is 0.5 mcg/kg/min, with a maximum of 10 mcg/kg/min. It is the paralytic of choice for patients with renal or hepatic insufficiency due to its minimal and transient side effects.

6. Ketamine

Ketamine is available at a concentration of 5 mg/mL and is used in variable doses depending on the clinical indication, such as induction, maintenance of anesthesia, status , or refractory pain management.

7. Morphine

Morphine, with a standard concentration of 1 mg/mL, is started at 0.2 mg/hr and increased to a maximum of 30 mg/hr. Reserved for severe pain unresponsive to other analgesics, it should be avoided in renal dysfunction due to the risk of respiratory depression.

8. Hydromorphone

Hydromorphone is administered at a concentration of 1 mg/mL, starting at 0.5 mg/hr and titrated up to 3 mg/hr. It is significantly more potent than morphine, requiring dose reductions in renal or hepatic impairment due to the risk of respiratory depression.

Cardiovascular Agents

1. Norepinephrine

A first-line vasopressor in most scenarios, norepinephrine is prepared at 32 mcg/mL and initiated at 2 mcg/min, with a maximum dose of 40 mcg/min. It requires central line administration, and phentolamine is the antidote for extravasation-related ischemia.

2. Vasopressin

Commonly used at a concentration of 0.2 units/mL, it is administered at a fixed rate of up to 2.4 units/hr without titration. It is often added as a second-line vasopressor when norepinephrine requirements exceed double-digit doses.

3. Phenylephrine

Phenylephrine, a pure alpha agonist, is used at a concentration of 400 mcg/mL, starting at 10 mcg/min and increasing to a maximum of 400 mcg/min. Central line administration is preferred, but it is not routinely recommended for septic shock.

4. Epinephrine

Epinephrine is available at 32 mcg/mL and is started at 1 mcg/min, with a maximum of 10 mcg/min. It is more commonly used in ACLS protocols and anaphylaxis (via IM administration). Central line infusion is recommended to avoid extravasation, which can be treated with phentolamine.

5. Dobutamine

This inotropic agent, administered at a concentration of 1000 mcg/mL, is started at 2.5 mcg/kg/min and can be titrated to a maximum of 20 mcg/kg/min. It is primarily used for inotropic support, although norepinephrine remains the first-line agent in cardiogenic shock.

6. Dopamine

Dopamine is prepared at 1600 mcg/mL, starting at 5 mcg/kg/min and increasing to a maximum of 20 mcg/kg/min. Its use in ICU settings is limited due to a higher risk of arrhythmias.

Additional Agents

Amiodarone: Used for ventricular tachycardia and atrial fibrillation, starting with a bolus followed by continuous infusion. It has complex pharmacokinetics and risks of pulmonary and hepatic toxicity.

Nitroprusside: Effective for hypertensive emergencies but carries a risk of cyanide toxicity and hypotension.

Insulin: IV insulin is the preferred agent for managing hyperglycemia and diabetic ketoacidosis in critical settings, requiring close monitoring of blood glucose and potassium.

These agents must be carefully monitored, with dosing adjustments as needed based on individual patient factors and clinical conditions.

Conclusion

This guide serves as a comprehensive resource for medical students, residents, and clinicians navigating the complexities of critical care, particularly within the ICU and pulmonary settings. Throughout the chapters, we have explored essential clinical practices, management protocols, and therapeutic approaches that are foundational to providing effective, evidence-based care in high-stress environments.

The initial chapters emphasized the importance of effective communication, timely interventions, and systematic documentation in the management of patients in both day and night MICU settings. The integration of interdisciplinary approaches, including consultations and transfers, alongside the meticulous management of consultations, patient readmissions, and documentation, is pivotal for smooth operations within the ICU. The clarity provided in the management of critical care emergencies, including sepsis, ARDS, and GI bleeding, underscores the need for swift action, precise diagnosis, and coordinated care efforts to optimize patient outcomes.

We also delved into the core aspects of mechanical ventilation and ventilator management, offering a detailed understanding of ventilation modes and settings, alongside the essential strategies for liberation from mechanical ventilation. These practices are crucial for ensuring patient comfort and minimizing long-term complications. The insights on chronic conditions such as COPD and asthma, as well as the management of life-threatening complications like DKA and HHS, reflect the complexity and interdisciplinary nature of critical care.

In addressing acid-base disorders and sedation practices, the guide reinforces the importance of precise diagnostics and individualized treatment approaches, enabling clinicians to navigate the fine balance between effective sedation and minimizing complications like delirium. The chapters also stress the role of pharmacological interventions, particularly the use of sedatives, analgesics, and paralytics, and the management of cardiovascular agents, in maintaining patient stability in the ICU.

Lastly, the understanding of delirium in critical care further highlights the need for proactive, patient-centered approaches in the ICU. By recognizing the signs, risk factors, and management strategies, clinicians can mitigate the impact of delirium, ultimately improving patient recovery and outcomes.

In conclusion, this book aims to equip healthcare providers with the essential tools and knowledge to deliver optimal care in the critical care setting. By integrating detailed clinical protocols, evidence-based treatment strategies, and a holistic approach to patient management, clinicians are empowered to face the challenges of the ICU with confidence, compassion, and expertise. Through continued education, collaboration, and a commitment to best practices, we can foster an environment where patient care and safety are the highest priorities.

References

1. Irwin & Rippe's Intensive Careers Medicine (8th Edition)

2. Marino's The ICU Book (4th Edition)

3. Oxford Handbook of Critical Care (3rd Edition)

4. Surviving Sepsis Campaign Guidelines (2021 Update)

5. ARDS Network Low Tidal Volume Study (2000)

6. Early Goal-Directed Therapy in Sepsis (Rivers et al., 2001)

7. American College of Chest Physicians (ACCP) Guidelines for Mechanical Ventilation

8. Critical Care Medicine Journal

9. Manual of ICU Procedures (2nd Edition)

10. Principles of Critical Care (4th Edition)

Glossary

1. **ABG (Arterial Blood Gas):** A test measuring oxygen, carbon dioxide, and pH levels in arterial blood, critical for assessing respiratory and metabolic function.

2. **ARDS (Acute Respiratory Distress Syndrome):** A severe inflammatory condition affecting the lungs, leading to impaired oxygenation.

3. **BP (Blood Pressure):** The pressure exerted by circulating blood upon the walls of blood vessels, essential for monitoring circulatory status.

4. **CVC (Central Venous Catheter):** A catheter placed into a large vein for medication delivery, fluid management, or hemodynamic monitoring.

5. **FiO$_2$ (Fraction of Inspired Oxygen):** The percentage of oxygen in the air mixture delivered to a patient, used to assess respiratory support.

6. **ICU (Intensive Care Unit):** A specialized unit providing advanced monitoring and life-sustaining treatments for critically ill patients.

7. **MAP (Mean Arterial Pressure):** The average arterial blood pressure during one cardiac cycle, vital for ensuring adequate organ perfusion.

8. **PEEP (Positive End-Expiratory Pressure):** A mechanical ventilation setting maintaining airway pressure above atmospheric levels to prevent alveolar collapse.

9. **Sepsis**: A life-threatening organ dysfunction caused by a dysregulated immune response to infection.

10. **Tidal Volume (VT):** The volume of air moved into or out of the lungs during a normal breath, crucial in mechanical ventilation.

11. **VAP (Ventilator-Associated Pneumonia):** A lung infection occurring in patients on mechanical ventilation for more than 48 hours.

12. **Vasopressors**: Medications used to constrict blood vessels and raise blood pressure in patients with shock.

13. **Weaning**: The gradual reduction of ventilator support to transition a patient to independent breathing.

14. **Critical Care Protocols:** Standardized guidelines used to manage common ICU conditions effectively and consistently.

15. **Hemodynamic Monitoring**: Techniques for measuring the blood flow and pressure within the cardiovascular system to guide clinical management.

16. **Acidosis**: A condition in which the body's fluids contain an excess of acid, often assessed through arterial blood gas analysis.

17. **Analgesia**: The absence of pain achieved through medication or other interventions, commonly used in ICU settings.

18. **Anuria**: The absence of urine production, often indicative of kidney failure or severe dehydration.

19. **Cardiac Output (CO):** The volume of blood the heart pumps per minute, critical for assessing cardiovascular function.

20. **Delirium**: Acute confusion or disorientation, frequently seen in critically ill patients and associated with prolonged ICU stays.

21. **DIC (Disseminated Intravascular Coagulation):** A severe condition causing widespread blood clotting and bleeding, often seen in sepsis or trauma.

22. **Endotracheal Tube (ETT):** A tube inserted into the trachea to provide an airway for mechanical ventilation.

23. **Enteral Nutrition**: Feeding provided through a tube directly into the gastrointestinal tract, essential for critically ill patients unable to eat orally.

24. **Hypercapnia:** Elevated carbon dioxide levels in the blood, often indicating respiratory insufficiency.

25. **Hypertension Crisis**: A severe increase in blood pressure that can lead to end-organ damage, requiring immediate intervention.

26. **Hypoxemia**: Low levels of oxygen in the blood, a common complication in critically ill patients.

27. **Ischemia**: Reduced blood flow to tissues, potentially leading to organ damage or failure.

28. **Multiorgan Dysfunction Syndrome (MODS):** The progressive failure of two or more organ systems in critically ill patients.

29. **Norepinephrine**: A vasopressor frequently used in critical care to treat septic shock and maintain blood pressure.

30. **Prone Positioning**: Placing a patient face down to improve oxygenation in severe respiratory failure, such as in ARDS.

31. **Sedation**: The use of medications to calm or induce sleep, commonly used to manage agitation in ventilated patients.

32. **Shock**: A life-threatening condition of inadequate blood flow to the tissues, requiring urgent management.

33. **Spontaneous Breathing Trial (SBT):** A test to determine whether a patient is ready to be weaned off mechanical ventilation.

34. **Swan-Ganz Catheter**: A device used to measure pressures in the heart and pulmonary arteries for advanced hemodynamic monitoring.

35. **Tracheostomy**: A surgical procedure to create a direct airway through an incision in the trachea, often used for prolonged ventilation.

36. **Vasoactive Medications**: Drugs that affect blood vessel tone, used to manage blood pressure and cardiac output in critical care.

37. **Work of Breathing (WOB):** The effort required to inhale and exhale, closely monitored in respiratory support patients.

38. **Zeroing**: The calibration of monitoring devices to ensure accurate hemodynamic readings in ICU settings.

www.ingramcontent.com/pod-product-compliance
Lightning Source LLC
Chambersburg PA
CBHW070351230526
45471CB00006B/2519